# Hair Loss

*A Comprehensive Guide on Prevention, Treatment and Hair Regrowth*

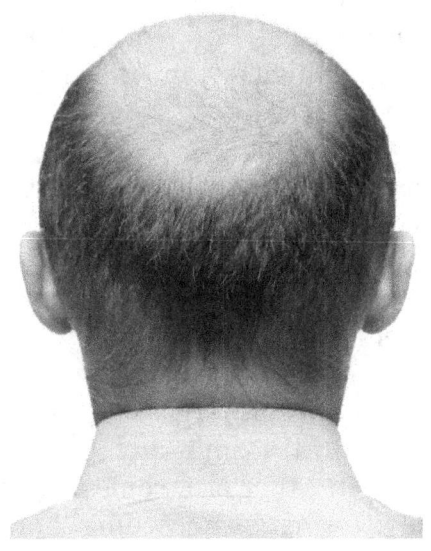

By

**Fhilcar Faunillan**

the owned by the owners themselves, not affiliated with this document.

# **Table of Contents**

# INTRODUCTION

Hello there reader! This is a good day for reading, is it not? Before digging deeper into the content of this book, first of all I would like to give you my hear felt gratitude for choosing to purchase and download my book, *"Hair Loss: A Comprehensive Guide on Prevention, Treatment and Hair Regrowth"*. Secondly, I would like to congratulate you for you are now in the possession of a book that would surely be beneficial to you. Clearly you need help concerning your hair or you know who does since you have this book. Do not worry. This book holds information that would certainly answer your queries.

Try to look around and look at everyone's head. Surely, you will find different types of people. You might be able to bump into someone who dyed their hair, wearing a headdress, having highlights, putting on too much gel and others. Yes, people are so diverse that we do things differently including those we want to do with our hair. If you would try and look a little bit harder you would find out that quite a few number of the male population is suffering from a middle life crisis. Most of them are going bald. Males who are belonging to the early 30s to the late 40s age bracket often experience thinning hairlines. A lot of them would have already lost eight percent of their total hair by the age of fifty. On the other hand, the female population has way more different hairstyles than that of the male counterpart. All of these styling and cutting would result to them having frizzy and unhealthy hair. The chemicals that women love so much to put in their hair are a huge contributing factor to their increasing hair falls and thinning hairlines.

This kind of thing is something that we thought is insignificant when we were young. We thought that since it is happening to most people, then it is not a big deal. We never worry about these kinds of things when we were young since they are way into the future. It is not until we experience it firsthand that we become conscious and alarmed about it. If you are reading this book then there is a high chance that you are suffering from this right now. While there is nothing to be so serious about it though since this is not a life threatening situation, this has caused low self-esteem and depression to many of the men who are faced with this problem. Always remember that there is a light at the end of every tunnel that we pass through. This is something that can be cured with the right remedy.

If you are a reader who is not yet suffering from hair loss then try to look at your parents and evaluate them. What age did they start losing their hair? Do they still have healthy hair right now? This might give you a heads up on what to expect on the days to come.

I have included here some steps and strategies on how to prevent, treat, and regrow your hair. To make things easier for you, I have also included some tips that you may follow in order to have the hair that you want and maybe deserve. So go and keep on reading in order to find out what these things may be. I do hope that you enjoy exploring all of its pages and learn through every page you turn.

Once again thank you for downloading this book and happy reading!

# Chapter 1 - All About Hair Loss

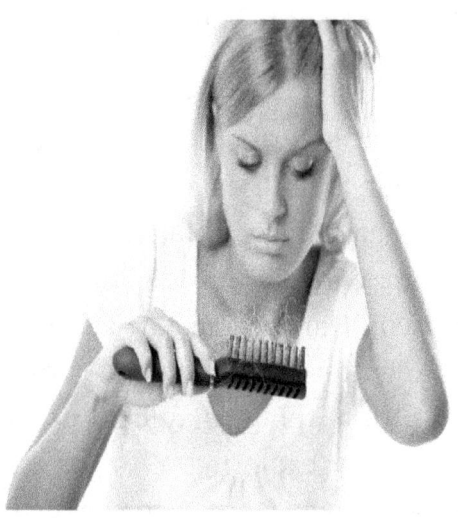

Hair grows everywhere in the human body. Except from the palms of our hands and the soles of our feet, you can pretty much find hair anywhere else. Keratin is what we call the protein that is used by our body to grow hair. As our body produces more hair cells, the old ones are being pushed out through the outer layer of skin which is what we see as hair. As a matter of fact, the hairs that we see are actually strings of old dead keratin cells. Science says that our hair grow at an average of six inches per year.

Don't you just hate it that every time you take a shower you see that your bathroom floor is full of your fallen hairs? Or when you are just casually combing it in front of a mirror and when you take a look at your comb, so many hairs has already been caught in its teeth? Or when you try and get yourself a haircut but your hair does not grow as fast as before or as thick as before?

Studies have shown that males are more likely to lose their hair than women. Most of these cases are caused because of male pattern baldness. However, thinning and losing hair is also common to women. This is the reason why there are so many cosmetic products available out there that is pledged to fight hair loss. This is not only common to women, it is also demoralizing.

It is true that in the world that we are living today, people are so obsessed in trying to look their best especially women. One way to project the beauty that they possess is through their hair. This is why having a great hair is so important to some of them. Researchers suggest that women who suffer from hair loss and thinning hair lines tend to become more insecure and have lower self-esteem. They become embarrassed about their condition.

As common as it may be treated, there are many reasons why hair loss is happening to you. Knowing the right source of your condition is the optimal way if you want to find the best cure for it. One of the major reasons why men suffer from hair loss as early as a teenager is because of male pattern baldness. This is a hereditary male condition where there is a receding hairline at the front of their heads or thinning hair at the top of their heads.

Androgenic Alopecia is the more scientific term of Male Pattern Baldness. This is more common and obvious to men than women. Males can suffer this condition as early as their teens and early 20s. On the other hand, females who suffer from this condition can experience and see noticeable thinning when they are already in their 40s. Males suffering from this can will experience the slow disappearance of their hair from the crown of their heads to the frontal area while females can see noticeable thinning at the crown of their heads.

What is causing this Male Pattern Baldness that is affecting almost 80% of the world's population? It is widely believed by scientists and researchers that this phenomenon is caused by a substance that is released inside our body and circulates throughout the system. This substance is called dihydrotestosterone or DHT. This is what causes for our hair follicle to shrink and lie dormant.

According to studies, this DHT is created by converting testosterone into this through an enzyme which is called 5a-reductase. Furthermore, these studies have shown that 5a-reductase is classified into two, Type 1 and Type 2. Type 1 covers only one-third of the total DHT circulating our body while Type 2 covers two-thirds. Type 1 can be found in the sebaceous glands of the skin including our hair while Type 2 5a-reductase is the enzyme that can be found at our hair follicles.

Research have shown that male having this male pattern baldness have scalps having small hair follicles and a greater amount of DHT compared to men who have lots of hair. Also, researchers have also found out that those males that possess 5a-reductase deficiency do not suffer from Male Pattern Hair Loss.

As exhausting as this may sound, this is only the tip of the iceberg. Aside from the hormones and enzymes that is being circulated in our body and aside from the inherited genes that we got from our parents, there are still a lot more external factors that we may be exposed to and are just neglecting them. Some of them may be included in our habits and some of them may be found in the environment where we live in. No matter how small or big the factor is, all of them can result to our decreasing chutzpah caused by this hair loss. To know what these factors are in order to prevent and treat them, I have listed here the causes of hair loss:

## 1. Physical Stress

When your body suffers from any physical trauma like an accident, surgery, severe illness, or even just the flu, this can cause for any hair loss. This kind of condition is called telogen effluvium. According to Marc Glashofer, a known dermatologist in New York City, here are three stages in the life cycle of your hair when you suffer from this. The first stage is the growth phase, and then followed by the rest phase and the last stage is the shedding phase. He also added that when your body has experienced a really stressful happening, this can shock your hair cycle which would put it into shedding phase a little bit longer. According to study, hair loss can become noticeable three to six months after the event. The good news is that your hair would start to grow again after your body has recovered. The faster you heal, the sooner would your hair can grow back.

## 2. Pulled-back Hair

This is a little quite significant among women but there is an increasing number of men out there who want their hair to be long. You should know that wearing hair in tight braids such as dreadlocks can affect the scalp and the way your hair would grow. In addition, having hair that is pulled back tightly, like those with ponytails, can lead to hair loss. In a more scientific term, this condition is known as traction alopecia. Since there is a continuous pulling of the hair, this will cause to a gradual hair loss especially on the hairline.

## 3. Pregnancy

Obviously this is only in the case of women. Pregnancy can be considered as a physical trauma which can lead to hair loss. This kind of hair loss is actually experienced after you have conceived your baby rather than during the pregnancy itself. When you are suffering from this, there is nothing to worry about since it is a normal scenario for women. Your hair would start to grow back after a couple of months.

### 4. Too Much Vitamin A

This is a testament to the saying, *"Too much is not good"*. Vitamin A gives our body the essentials needed like better vision, but just like anything else, an excess of this substance is not good for our body. According to the American Academy of Dermatology, our daily intake of Vitamin A should 5,000 International Units (IU) per day for adults. Supplements of kids over the age of four can contain 2,500 to 10,000 IU. Fortunately, this is a reversible condition. Once your body has exhausted all of the extra Vitamin A in your body, your hair would regrow.

## 5. Lack of Protein

If too much Vitamin A can cause hair loss, then not enough protein can cause it too. If your body does not have enough protein intakes, then it can ration protein from another source. One way that our body can do this is by shutting down hair growth in order for it to have a more ample supply of protein. They say that this can take place about two to three months after the drop in your protein diet.

## 6. Female Hormones

Just like the fact that pregnancy can cause hair loss, so thus the change in the hormonal release of the body of the females. This kind of situation usually takes place when they first try or stop using birth control. Female should be aware that taking contraceptives such as birth pills can cause disturbance to the

19

hormonal balance of our body. This change in the equilibrium would also become more evident and more likely to happen if your family has a history of hair loss. Also, when women undergo menopause, they also have hormonal changes in their body. This too can cause hair loss or telogen effluvium. One way to prevent this is to switch birth control pills. Of course, it would be safer if you would consult a doctor about the different types of contraceptives.

## 7. Trichotillomania

This is classified by experts as a behavioral action. It is still unclear whether to classify it as a habit or under the category of obsessive-compulsive disorder. One thing is for sure though, it can cause hair loss. This Trichotillomania is the more scientific term of the behavioral disorder wherein people having this have the need to always pluck or pull their hair. It does not matter whether it is the hair on their head, arms or legs. The important thing for them is that they are able to ease their longing to pluck some hair. Over time, this might cause some wound to a certain area which can later be transformed into a scar. This scar would prevent the growth of hair which would be the common cause of a bald spot in our hair. If a certain person who has this condition would stop the soonest time possible, hair regrowth can also be possible over time. However, if this continues for a long time, this can lead to permanent hair loss on the affected area.

## 8. Anemia

According to studies, one in about ten people suffer from anemia which can become a cause of hair loss. The most common source of this ailment is due to the lack of iron in the body. This is really common to women aged 20 through 50. The doctor can run some tests on your blood in order to be sure if you have this kind of anemia. If it turns out to be positive, then just a little change in your diet and some supplement intake can reverse its effects. This is one source of hair loss that is really easy to cure.

## 9. Hypothyroidism

The thyroid is a small organ that can be found at the front of our neck just below the voice box. This small gland releases hormones that are critical to our body's metabolism. Since it plays an important role to our metabolism, it controls our body's growth and development. In certain conditions when our thyroid is not pumping out enough hormones sufficient for our body, it might affect our development including hair growth. Hypothyroidism or underactive thyroid gland can be caused by some abnormalities brought about by birth, some autoimmune deficiencies or surgery which includes the removal of the thyroid gland. Fortunately, the future is now better thanks to science. Synthetic Thyroid medication is available which then has the effect of returning the thyroid hormone level back to normal.

## 10. Vitamin B Deficiency

Just like Vitamin A, our body can also suffer from hair loss if we lack Vitamin B in our system. Although this is not a common cause of hair loss, in some rare cases, this can cause hair loss. The good news however is that, this is so correctible. Like anemia and Vitamin A deficiency, simple supplementation and proper diet would solve your problem.

You can find Vitamin B on foods like fish, meat, vegetables, and non-citrus fruits.

## 11. Autoimmune Diseases

Autoimmune-related hair loss can be caused not only by poor immune system but only when it is overly active. This condition is also known as alopecia areata. This occurs when our body gets confused. The immune system sees the hair as something foreign or alien and attacks it. Other types of this disease are diabetes or arthritis, when our body attacks healthy body tissues. When this happens on our hair follicle, it can cause cicatrical alopecia or permanent hair loss and telogen effluvium or temporary disruption of hair growth. You can take some medications in order to alter this.

## 12. Infections

There are a lot of infections that can cause hair loss. The most common infection that can affect our scalp and hair follicles is that which is caused by ringworms. What many people think is that ringworms are actually worms. This is not the case. Do not let the name fool you. Ringworm infection is actually caused by fungus. This type of condition is more scientifically known as the Tinea capitis. This is due to mold-like fungi called dermophytes. The favorite habitat of these fungi are warm moist places which can happen to our hair if we practice poor hygiene. This is more common to children but adults can also catch this.

## 13. Chemotherapy

This is the number one treatment know for cancer patients. Cancer cells are dangerous cells that divide and grow faster than the body's healthy cells. The reason why chemotherapy is so effective in treating cancer is that it stops these cells to grow rapidly. The bad news is that cancer cells are not the only cells that grow rapidly in our body. Another group of cells that grow rapidly can be found in our hair follicles. When our body is exposed to radiation which is caused by chemotherapy, it does not only destroy cancer cells but hair cells as well. The hair would regrow once you are no longer exposed to chemotherapy's radiation.

## 14. Dramatic Weight Loss

You might want to lose a lot of pounds that is why you starve yourself or you stress your body by working out too much, but this kind of practice is not healthy. The road to fitness is not something that you can go to through shortcut without harming yourself. It takes time to be perfectly and physically fit. When you starve yourself, your body does not gain the vitamins and minerals that it needs in order to function properly. Also, when you exhaust your body too much, this might cause a physical trauma. Both of these can cause hair loss. Losing hair and body weight at the same time are both symptoms of eating disorders like anorexia or bulimia.

## 15. Polycystic Ovary Syndrome

Obviously, this only affects women. POS is a condition wherein there is an imbalance between the male and female sex hormones. Studies have shown that having too much androgen have many side effects which includes: infertility, irregular menstrual cycle, weight gain, ovarian cyst and hair thinning. Sometimes when male hormones are too present, a woman can grow hair on her face and on her body.

## 16. Medications

Some medications can help correct the reasons why you are losing your hair but there are some out there which may cause the opposite effect of what you want to achieve. Some common drugs that have hair thinning as a side effect are antidepressants and blood thinners. Other drugs that might cause hair loss are lithium, methotrexate (used in curing rheumatic and skin ailments), anti-inflammatory drugs including ibuprofen and others. Consult your doctor about the medications that you are taking. If you have discovered that it is causing the thinning of your hair then ask him to lower the dosage or switch to other drugs.

## 17. Over styling

Braids and ponytails are not the only cause of thinning hair. Sometimes when you want to look your best, you tend to find the best hairstyle that would suite you. This can become a trial and error process which would include lots and lots of hair cosmetics like wax, gel, hairspray, and dye among others. This can irritate you scalp which would then result to a receding hairline. In addition, technologies like hot-oil, rebonding and perming can damage our hair. When our hair is exposed to high heat or harsh chemicals, sometimes they affect not only the tip of our hair but also down to its roots. If the roots are damaged, your hair might not just grow back.

## 18. Aging

Aging is something inevitable. Whether we like it or not, we are all going to grow old. When we grow old, so do our bodies including our hair follicles. When this happens, hair regeneration may not be like before. When women reach the age of forty or fifty, hair degeneration becomes quite obvious. Experts are not really sure why this is happening. This is the reason why people would settle for wigs, scarves and hair styles that would cover up the thin areas.

## 19. Anabolic Steroids

According to American Academy of Dermatology, taking anabolic steroids would result to hair loss. This is an alarming situation for athletes since they tend to abuse this stuff in order to gain more muscle and strength. Researches have shown that taking anabolic steroids have the same effect as having polycystic ovary disease. The best way to cure this is to go off the drug.

# Chapter 2 - How to Prevent Hair Loss

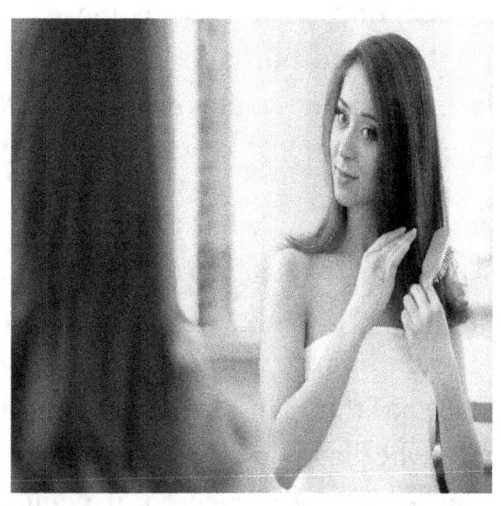

Every day, everyone loses hair in their head. To iterate, there is no need to freak out since this is a natural occurrence. Hair is continuously growing and when some strands have reached the tip of their life cycle, they fall and are being replaced by other strands. But when we are talking about inherited male pattern baldness, it means that there are fewer strands of hair growing which is not enough to compensate to the number of the fallen ones. In a research conducted by the American Hair Loss Association, it was found that two-thirds of the American male population would experience hair loss by the age of 35.

Now that we know what are causing hair loss, one way to make sure that we do not suffer from this in the future is to know what to do in order for us to be prepared in fighting this kind of condition. For people who have suffered from hair loss and have already recovered, it would be best to keep in your mind that there is more than one way in order for you to experience hair loss once again.

Yes, the good news is that there are numerous ways in order to prevent hair loss. Women more often neglect these ways since hair loss is not so much obvious until they reach a certain age. However, researches have shown that one third of the world's population are suffering from hair loss. From that given fraction, thousands are women. Just like what have been discussed in the previous chapter, there are multiple causes of hair loss, including vitamin deficiencies, diet, medications, stress and genetics. Of all these reasons, genes is the number one cause of hair loss especially to men.

When it comes to prevention, there is no surefire guarantee that hair loss can be inhibited when it is genetically programmed. If you observe and see your parents suffer from hair loss caused by aging, then there is a good chance that you too would suffer from it as you grow older. Nevertheless, there are still some ways on how to slow down this aging or hair loss. You can stop the source of whatever it is that is causing your head to lose hair at a fast rate. You can always follow certain procedures and rules in order for you to enjoy your hair for as long as you can.

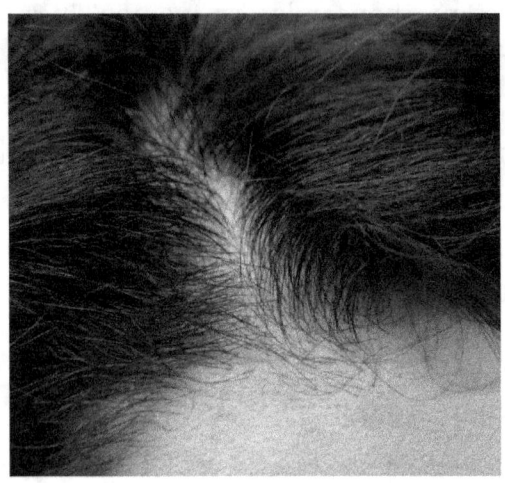

*Here are some ways that you can do in order to prevent hair loss:*

1. **Find the source.** For you to find the right cure, the first step is to know what the cause is. You can never address you hair loss dilemma properly unless you point out the source of it. Say, you cannot get away from your hair loss if the cause of it is your medication but the cure you

34

are doing is by eating more healthy foods. Your hair loss would still be there since you are still taking into your body the cause of it. The only way to prevent it is by changing medications. Doctors diagnose balding through sight mostly. If your head is losing hair on the sides and middle top of it, this is mostly the cause of male pattern baldness. While if the thinning of the hair happens throughout the scalp indicates some underlying health issues. Marc Avram of Weill Cornell Medical College said to never assume that every hair loss is caused by genes.

2. **Go natural.** One way that we lose our hair is because of the cosmetics and products that we are so fond of applying on our hair. Also, different hair stylings put our hair in harsh conditions which can cause for it to give in and fall. What you can do is to stay away from all these

products. Do not color your hair if you can in order for it to have its natural color. Do not straighten or curl your hair. Let it flow the way it should be. Not touching your hair would cause less damage to your hair since you are letting it grow on its own life cycle. However, if not touching your hair is not an option for you, you can always give your hair some time to recover from the damage that it has suffered due to blowouts and chemical treatments.

3. **Limit yourself from using hair dryers.** The hair dryer or blower is one of the most commonly used accessories for the hair. It is used not only to dry the hair but also to style it. The immediate cause of this habit is breakage since your hair would become more brittle making it prone to damage. Hair dryers work because they emit heat. Heat weakens proteins. Without protein, our hair would

become more fragile which would lead to hair loss that would have not occurred otherwise. Natural drying is best for your hair, so if you have the time, let your hair dry naturally than using your blowers more often.

4. **Other hair devices can damage your hair.** Hair dryers or blowers are not the only things that can destroy our scalp. Other devices like hair curlers, hair straighteners and hot brushes also have the same effect as hair dryers. If you do not have any choice but to use these devices, then always give your hair some time to recover from the damage that it has dealt before. In addition, be very careful when using heated devices since burnt scalps can cause permanently damaged hair follicles.

5. **Avoid Perming and bleaching your hair.** Perming refers to either straightening or curling your hair. These two can both destroy your hair. Perming works because it breaks the inner bonds of the hair in order to straighten or curl it. On the other hand, bleaching your hair removes the natural pigment present in our hair. This happens because cuticles are being penetrated by chemicals. This too can change the structure of the hair, making it more prone to damage. Both of these can contribute to hair loss later.

6. **Switch shampoos.** Many shampoo commercials claim that their product would make your hair thicker and healthier. However, according to studies, only one ingredient is proven to preserve your scalp which is called Ketoconazole. This is an antifungal ingredient which is used to fight dandruff. This can save your pate since it would help reduce the

production of testosterone, therefore DHT, in hair follicles. A Belgian study has proven that balding men who used a shampoo with Ketoconazole two or three times a week for half a year saw a 17 percent reduction in their hair loss.

7. **Hot oil treatments.** This does not mean that you have to go to a salon. Most salons engage in technology to do their service. Most of these technologies can damage your hair. Do it more naturally. You can take any natural oil – coconut, olive, or canola – and heat it up. Be sure to check the temperature of the oil before applying it to your hair. When the temperature is just right, massage it gently into your head. Put on a shower cap and leave it there for an hour. Rinse afterwards using shampoo. You can also find some substitute for oils by using natural juices like garlic juice, onion juice or ginger juice. They require to be

lathered thoroughly and be left overnight. You can wash it thoroughly in the morning.

8. **Care for your hair actively.** Having proper hygiene is one way to stay away from conditions that can cause hair loss. By always taking good care of your hair, you can reduce the chances of having hair loss at a notch. One way to care for your hair is by washing it regularly with mild shampoo. This would clean your hair which would reduce the chances of having some infections and diseases that would affect your scalp and hair follicles. Find the perfect shampoo for you. Using the most suitable shampoo for your hair would make it grow healthier and thicker.

9. **Try scalp massage.** A head or scalp massage would increase the blood flow to the surface of your skin. This would result

to a better circulation of nutrients and mineral for your scalp and hair follicles. Scalp massage is usually accompanied by egg oil in order to maximize hair growth potential but anything else works. In addition, a head massage would help you distress which would result to a better overall body function.

10. **Brush your hair properly.** How you brush can either break or make your hair. Contrary to what others do mostly when they comb their hair, the right way to brush your hair is not from top to down but from inside out. When you brush your hair, be as gentle as you can be. Do not pull really hard. Also, find the perfect comb for you. Do not settle for the cheap ones you can find for they have harsh bristles. Buy hairbrush or combs that are made of natural fibers. Always remember to never brush your hair when it is wet since this is the time when our hair is

most fragile. Use comb when you have to deal with wet hair.

11. **Test your hair if you are concerned about hair loss.** You can know whether you are suffering from hair loss by doing a little test known as the "tug" test. This is done by taking a small group of your hair, about 20-30 strands, and holding them firmly between your thumb and index finger. Pull slowly but firmly. If there are more six or more than six hairs that came out at the same time, you may be suffering from hair loss. This is not a fool-proof test so if you think that you are losing hair than usual, be sure to check on your doctor.

12. **Use antioxidants.** Apply warm green tea on your hour. Just like hot oil treatments, leave it for like an hour before rinsing. Green tea contains antioxidants

which is not only good for our body but also for our hair. Antioxidants prevent hair loss by making our hair healthier and boosting hair growth.

13. **Meditate.** As what we have learned in the previous chapter, physical trauma and stress can sometimes cause hair loss. When our body is shocked due to sudden physical activity and exhaustion, this may trigger hair loss. Studies have shown that stress and tension is the cause of hair loss most of the time especially for women. Meditating would help your body to relax. Meditating exercises like Yoga and Pilates can help reduce and restore imbalance in our hormones.

14. **Eat Smarter.** It is due to malnutrition that we sometimes suffer from hair loss. If our body is not being nourished with enough vitamins and minerals, it would

inhibit the growth of our body including our hair. Our body would find other source of the nourishment that it needs that sometimes it takes up the nourishment that our body had reserved for hair regrowth. Here are some ways on how to improve your food intake which would have a great impact on the condition of your hair:

• **Have a healthy balanced diet –** Needless to say, having a healthy balanced diet would make not only your hair be in good condition but it works wonders on the entire whole body too. It is common sense that eating the right food would nourish your scalp and hair follicle which would then prevent hair loss. If you have a healthy body, having a healthy hair will soon follow. Having a healthy diet can also become as a factor that would slow down hair loss if you have gained it genetically. So be sure to eat healthily if you want to have a healthy hair.

• **Consume food that contain lots of Vitamin B6, Vitamin B12 and Folic Acid.** These three vitamins that fall under the B complex classification are all essential in the creation of hemoglobin in our blood. This hemoglobin is critical since it carries the needed oxygen from our lungs to different tissues in our body including the hair. Healthy hair strongly relies on ample supply of oxygen and blood. This is why head and scalp massage are effective ways to stimulate blood circulation to our head. If you have Vitamin B deficiency, it would be the same like cutting off blood supply in your hair which then lead to hair loss and slow hair regrowth.

• **Eat foods with lots of iron.** Iron is an essential food nutrient that we need in our body. Heme iron is the iron you get from animal sources while non-heme iron is that which can be found in plant sources. Iron helps develop red blood cells in the system; having too little of these would lead to anemia. If you have anemia, nutrient-flow is being disrupted thus your hair follicles could not regenerate the way it used to be. To avoid this, make sure to eat iron-rich foods like red meat, fish and chicken. Good sources of non-heme iron are green vegetables like spinach and broccoli.

• **Have enough protein intakes.** Protein is what primarily makes up our hair, so it just makes sense to eat a lot of food which are rich with protein in order to continuously nourish our hair. If you have protein deficiency, your hair follicle could not efficiently function which then results to more hair loss than hair regrowth. Also, without proper protein intake would result to weak and dry hair. There are shampoos that claim to have protein as an active ingredient. This might help, but it is the protein in our diet that has the greatest impact to our overall hair health. It is known to almost everyone that meat is a rich source of protein. Words of caution though, do not try to eat steak every day since this would not help you. Foods like steak contain high amounts of fat which would result to an increase to your testosterone level. We have discussed it in the previous chapters that testosterone can lead to hair loss, thus, steak does not belong to the food group that helps prevent hair loss. Stick to leaner meat on your diet which includes fish, chicken, soy milk, cheese, eggs, beans, almonds, peanut butter and nuts.

• **Have enough Vitamin C intake.** What most people do not know is that Vitamin C helps in the good absorption of iron. The best way to get the most of the iron on food intakes would be by combining iron-rich foods with those foods which have high Vitamin C content in them. Vitamin C is also essential in producing collagen that is good for the capillaries in our hair follicles. These collagens are the connective tissue that holds tissues in the body, in this case the hair shafts. People get most of their Vitamin C intake on citrus foods. However, there are more foods that can give us Vitamin C which includes green leafy vegetables, tomatoes, peppers, salad, baked potatoes, blueberries, blackberries and strawberries.

• **Be sure to get enough Omega-3 fatty acids.** These are fats that are good for your health unlike those that you can find in steaks. Not only are they good for your heart, they also play a vital role in keeping your hair healthy. These fats are found in the cells on your scalp and they keep it hydrated. Be sure to eat food that have these fats because they can only be obtained through food since our body could not produce these. A good source of this nutrient is through the consumption oily fish like salmon, tuna and mackerel. Other sources would be seeds and nuts like pumpkin seeds and walnuts.

• **You can take supplements.** Supplements are different from the usual medications since they do not cure any disease. They just give your body the nutrients that it needs in order to function properly. You should only take supplements that are approved by the FDA and other authorized agencies. In order to be sure, you can talk to your medical practitioner bout your needs. As him or her what is the best supplement for you to take in order to prevent hair loss. There are a lot of supplements that can fight hair loss. When you inquire about it you should consider finding supplements which include biotin, vitamin C, iron, inositol and palmetto.

• **Drink lots of water.** Keeping yourself hydrated is one key factor in maintaining good health. Seventy percent of our body is made up of water which means that every cell and organ in our body uses water in order to function properly. It is not enough to just wash your hair with water; you should also nourish it by drinking lots of it. Not having enough water in your body can lead to poor nutrition which can lead to other diseases like anorexia. Anorexia can lead to severe malnutrition which would trigger the hair follicle to stop their growth cycle. Poor nutrition can also cause dramatic weight loss which can also trigger hair loss. Participating on an unhealthy diet can cause malnutrition which would result to imbalances in the body which can lead to hair loss. This is why water is so important to every living creature.

- **Know what not to eat.** Eating unhealthy and healthy foods at the same time can negate the nutritional benefits of it all. When you are trying to eat healthy, then stick with it and stay away from the unhealthy ones. It can sometimes be tempting to eat those greasy foods but consistency is vital. Basic rules apply when having a healthy balanced diet, however be very sure of the ingredients included to what you are eating. For example, the artificial food sweetener, aspartame, has been found out to contribute to hair thinning and hair loss. Food additives and foods with lots of preservatives also have a negative effect on our hair's health. Try to have the right amount of calories when eating since a low-calorie diet can deplete your energy which can also cause hair loss.

# Chapter 3 - How to Treat Hair Loss

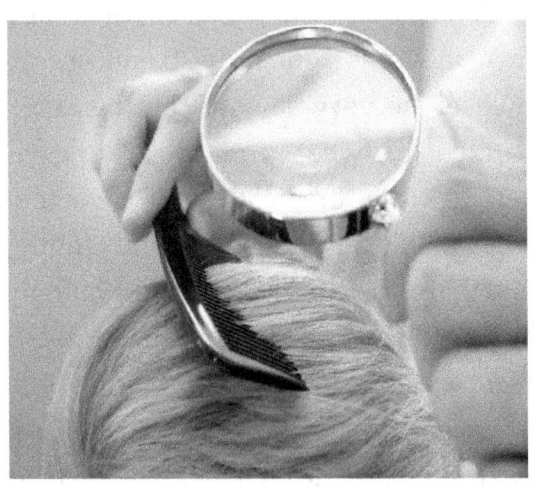

It is one thing to prevent hair loss and it is another when you try to treat it. Prevention is better than cure they say, I guess I have to agree with it. It would save you the time and effort if the disease did not happen in your body in the first place. However, no matter how much we want to never encounter diseases again in our entire life, this is not the case. Life will always give us struggles and one of these struggles would be ailments and conditions that we should overcome. A way of overcoming these ailments and conditions would be through treatment. Since it would be too late to prevent it, what you can do is to cure yourself from it and do your best to never suffer from the same disease again.

Hair Loss is one type of condition that we can prevent from happening. Some people however, discover that they are suffering from hair loss a little too late to prevent it. What you can do instead is to treat it. There are many ways on how to do this. Depending on the cause of hair loss, there are many options on what to do in order to treat the further shedding of your hair from your head. Certain treatments may involve minor efforts but in some cases, surgical and medical interventions might be needed.

In order for you to know the different treatments that can be used in order to heal hair loss, I have put here a list of things which you can do. Some of them are so easy that you can do them even at home. With the right ingredients and procedure, you can make your own homemade hair loss treatment. Here are ways on how to treat hair loss:

## 1. Visit your doctor.

When you think that your hair loss is caused by a more serious medical condition, then you should know when to give your doctor a visit. On most cases, hair loss is easily corrected if diagnosed properly. Some medical conditions that can cause temporary or permanent hair loss include: thyroid deficiency, autoimmune disorders, diabetes, lupus, trichotillomania, physical stress, anemia and other infections.

If you think that you are losing your hair rapidly or in an unusual pattern, then it would be best if you would consult your doctor. Other symptoms that you should consider being checked up by your doctor would include: Pain and itching with hair loss, red scalps and bald spots. When you do visit your doctor, you should prepare for your appointment. You should not be shy and tell the doctor everything that you have experienced including the first time when you experience the hair loss.

## 2.  Know the treatment for men.

In men, hereditary hair loss is the most common reasons for shedding off or even balding. You can recognize this since your receding hairline would create a letter "M" shape on your head. Although it is not a disease and are based on your genes, there are still some treatments that doctors can prescribe for you. There are two medications that doctors widely prescribed and these are applicable worldwide:

- Minoxidil – this is available as a lotion that you can apply on your scalp every day. You can easily buy them over-the-counter and there is no prescription is needed. There is no clear reason on how minoxidil works but there are some testimonies and evidence that show it clearly works. There are two types of these medications; either it contains 2% or 5% minoxidil. It is suggested that minoxidil (5%) is more effective than the one containing lesser percentage. However, it may cause more side effects like dryness and itchiness to the area where it is applied. Do not be dismayed if you do not see any immediate results after you have applied this lotion. It usually takes several months before any evident result can be seen. It is also said that hair thinning would resume once you have stopped using this medication. Any new hair that grows would shed after two months of withdrawal from minoxidil. Do not worry because side effects just happen on rare occasions.

- Finasteride – This medication can only be bought if you have been given a private prescription by your physician. Finasteride comes in the form of a tablet that you take every day. This product works by preventing testosterones to be converted into dihydrotestosterone (DHT). As what have been said in the previous chapters, DHT promotes hair loss by shrinking the hair follicles. Finasteride makes sure that they go back to their normal size. There are also many testimonies and evidences which prove that Finasteride works. Just like minoxidil, it usually takes three to six months of continuous medication before any evident result can be obviously seen. The balding process would also resume six to twelve months after you have stopped taking the medication. Just like minoxidil, Finasteride's side effects are uncommon. According to research, less than 1 in 100 men who take Finasteride has suffered from loss in sex drive and erectile dysfunction.

### 3. Know the treatment for women.

About one-third of the female population experience hair loss at some point of their lives. And two-thirds of women who are menopausal suffer from hair shedding and thinning. It is not common for women to have receding hairlines but what is common for them is the thinning of the hair on the top part of the hair. One kind of treatment for women would be minoxidil too which is applied onto the scalp. This can also be used in treating female pattern baldness. Studies have shown that women respond better to minoxidil than men. It usually takes lesser time for women to see any evident result as compared to men. Iron supplements are usually prescribed to most women, especially to vegetarians and those that have history of anemia. On some rare cases, anti-androgens are being prescribed to women. Anti-androgens are receptor-blocking drugs that help hair follicles to become healthy.

## 4. Be open to other treatment options

Another way to treat hair baldness is through transplant. Hair transplant is done by removing healthy hair follicles in your hair and putting them on areas where hair loss is most evident. Before doing this, consult a hair transplant surgeon. Ask him or her about the requirements needed in order to qualify for this operation. Also, ask him or her about the procedure including all of its possible side effects and cost. This type of procedure would involve the removal of hundreds of hair follicles which is a very hard thing to do which is why this procedure is usually so expensive. However, if you can afford such operations, the results are really excellent and permanent.

Another optional treatment in which you can venture into is called low-level light therapy. LLLT was discovered during the 1960s and is found to be abruptly helpful in healing wounds. Ask experts about products that use LLLT. Many of these products are approved by the FDA. Many patients who have undergone this treatment testified that they see positive results. While the mechanism beneath this LLLT is not yet fully understood, researches have indicated that this procedure would have effect on the cellular level which would improve hair growth on people. Studies are still being held right now in order to have a full understanding on the underlying mechanism behind this cure.

Melatonin is another way of treating hair loss patients. Ask your doctor about it. One research study has done an experiment on a small group of women who are all suffering from hair thinning. They all showed positive results when melatonin was used. Topical lavender is also another substance which is used in promoting hair growth. A study has also shown positive result in using lavender as the catalyst for hair regrowth. Take note that lavender should not be taken orally but should be applied on the scalp.

Immunotherapy is becoming a popular treatment for hair loss. This kind of treatment is most effective on people who already have extensive hair loss. Many people are taking their chances in this treatment even if only about half of those people who have undergone this procedure have seen promising results. This procedure is done by the use of a chemical solution called diphencyprone

(DPCP) which is applied to the area where hair loss can be seen. This is repeated every week with a higher dosage each time. Eventually, the chemical solution would lead the person to have an allergic reaction. On some cases, this will trigger hair regrowth after about 4 months. The possible side effects associated with this treatment may include extreme skin reaction, rash and vitiligo. Hair loss would eventually resume once this treatment is stopped. This kind of treatment is only available on specialized centers. This procedure would require you to wear a hat or scarf over the applied area in order for the light not to react with the chemical.

When you have been diagnosed with Alopecia areata, know that there are no hundred percent guarantees that there would be a completely effective way to treat it. One way to cure this is through Corticosteroids injections. This kind of injection contains steroids which is a hormone that is present in our body. This works since steroids suppress the immune system of the person being injected with it. This is really effective when it comes to treating Alopecia areata since this is a kind of hair condition wherein the immune system is the damaging the hair follicles. Corticosteroids are used not only on the scalp of our head but also on eyebrows. It is effective on healing small patches that are hairless. Just like other types of medications, alopecia might return once treatment has been stopped.

Tattooing can be used on people who would want to replicate their hair. This is also known as dermatography. Surprisingly during its introduction period, it has already gathered positive feedbacks among people who have their hair replicated. The downside of this procedure is that it is really expensive and can only be used in replicating really short hair. This is why dermatography is usually done on eyebrows and on males who are suffering from male pattern baldness.

Since tattoos can only be used to treat very short hair, people who have extensive hair loss can settle to wigs to cover up the affected area. Synthetic wigs are the cheapest wigs since they are made of acrylic. Their price ranges from 30-300 euros. Acrylic wigs can last up to nine months and is commonly found since they do not need a lot of styling. Their downside is that they are really hot to wear and can cause some itches on your head. Another type of wig which is used to cover up baldness are wigs which are made from real hair. Most people would prefer looking for these rather than the synthetic ones even if their price ranges are quite hefty. Real hair wigs are more comfortable to use but they should also be maintained highly. They require more attention since they should be styled and professionally cleaned to maintain its volume and beauty. If maintained properly, it can last for three to four years.

The latest treatment that has been discovered by experts that would be used in order to treat hair loss would be cloning. This technique involves the taking a little of the remaining hair cells of the person being treated, multiplying them and planting them into the bald areas of the head. The mechanics is a little bit the same with hair transplant but instead of using present hair currently, they would just clone the cells of the few ones left. Cloning can both be used to cure male- and female- hair pattern baldness. However, more studies should be conducted in order to assess the effectiveness of such procedure.

## 5. Try some home remedies.

If you have already seen the start of your hair fall, there are some things that you can do in order for you to prevent further damage even when you are at home. Sometimes our body can experience some side-effects from the chemical reactions which have been caused by some hair loss medications. Hair fall treatment at home can sometimes be what other people are looking for if they want to stay away from the harsh side effects of chemicals and medications. Always remember that it is normal for you to lose 50-100 strands of hair every day. That is not something alarming. But if you are losing more than that, maybe it is time for you to intervene and prevent it from becoming extensive.

*Here are some things that you can do when you are at home that are guaranteed to stop or slow down hair loss:*

- **Coconut**

o   Coconut is also known as the tree of life since all of its parts can be used for something. Well, one thing is that it can be used for is for treating hair loss. Coconut can become a very good source of many nutrients like good fats, proteins, potassium and iron which can all help in hair regrowth. You can either use coconut oil or coconut milk directly on your hair. Heat the coconut milk and leave it wrapped with a shower cap for a few hours before rinsing.

- **Onion Juice**

o   Onion is known to make people cry. In this particular case, it would make you smile since it can promote hair regrowth. Onion is a very good source of sulphur which is essential in increasing collagen production in our hair. Collagens are vital to hair regrowth since they connect hair to the follicles in order to get the most nutrients available. To apply, squeeze a fresh raw onion on your scalp and gently massage to stimulate deep into the roots. Leave it for an hour and finish off with your shampoo and conditioner. Applying this treatment regularly can work miracles.

- **Garlic**

o   Garlic is also the same with onion; it has a very rich amount of sulphur content which we all know is essential for hair regrowth. It is not surprising that garlic has been already used in the olden times as a traditional hair regime. Not only does it make hair regrow, it also has a lot more beauty benefits. Unlike onion, garlic treatment should be left overnight. Have a clove of garlic and gently apply on the affected area. After an hour, massage your scalp with olive oil. Rinse your hair and finish it off with your shampoo the following day.

- **Henna**

o   Henna is more known to be a natural hair color or as a conditioner, but henna have some substances that can promote hair regrowth by strengthening the roots of the hair. You can achieve your best hair by combining henna with other types of hair strengthening treatments.

- **Hibiscus**

o   This is also known as the shoe flower. Hibiscuses have properties that can prevent premature greying of the hair. It is also proven to be an effective ingredient in fighting dandruffs. In addition to that, hibiscus nourishes hair which can control hair fall.

- **Indian Gooseberry**

o   This is also known as the amla. People treat amla or Indian Gooseberries as blessings sent down from heaven above since it is really full of Vitamin C and antioxidants which can reverse hair fall. It would be best to apply gooseberry to your scalp if the hair loss is still on its initial stage.

- **Egg**

○ Eggs are really delicious and easy to cook. This is the reason why almost all households have eggs present in their fridge. Eggs is packed with several ingredients that can help hair to regrow and can help stop hair loss. Eggs contain active ingredients like sulphur, protein, phosphorous, selenium, iodine and zinc. All of these can promote hair regrowth. Egg works best as a conditioner and should be mixed thoroughly with olive oil. Apply it during your regular bath and utilize a shower cap after you you're your shampoo. Leave it on for about 10-20 minutes, rinse and apply a moisturizing conditioner then rinse again.

# Chapter 4 - Tips on How to Prevent/Treat Hair Loss and Maintain Healthy Hair

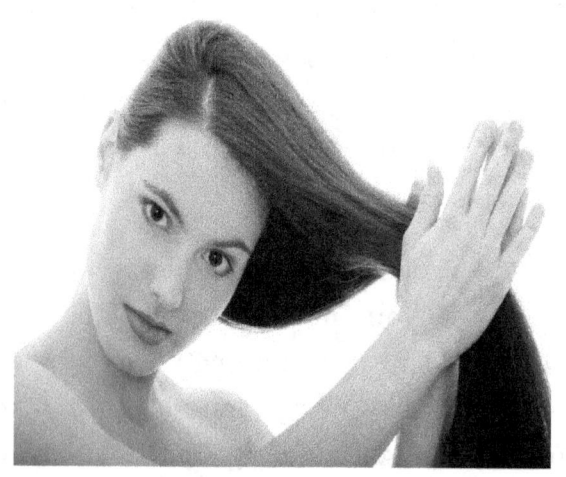

*Here are some tips in order to make your journey towards healthy scalp a little bit easier:*

• Sunlight is good for your skin since it would provide you with Vitamin D. However, avoid too much exposure of your hair to it since it can be damaging.

- Choose mild shampoo over anything else. Harsh chemicals would do no good on your hair.

- Keep yourself on a good condition. Exercise regularly. Illnesses and medications can cause hair loss which is why it would be best to keep yourself on a healthy condition to counter the effect of hair loss.

- If you just conceived a baby, do not worry if you suffer from postpartum alopecia. This is something normal for all mothers out there. Hair loss can be frightening during pregnancy but is all due to the hormonal changes caused by your pregnancy.

- Always wash your hair with gentleness. Do the same when brushing it.

- Always balance your nutrition. Eat lots of healthy foods.

- If you can, use natural products on your hair.

- Damaged hair is almost impossible to repair. What you can do is to have a haircut. Do not be discouraged if you lose few inches since it will grow back. Just focus on keeping the rest of your hair healthy until it grows back to your desired length.

- There is no such thing as a shampoo that can fix a spilt end. The only way to get rid of split ends is to trim it.

- Be very careful when you want to take pills and other kind of medications. To be sure, always consult your general physician before taking in anything in your body.

- Protect hair when swimming. Chlorine is a really harsh chemical which can result to heavy damage on your hair. This is why it would be best to wet and condition your hair before diving in. It would be

better if you can wear really tight swim
cap.

## Conclusion

I would like to congratulate you for being able to reach the last part of this book. Also, I would like to thank you again for choosing to purchase this book.

I do hope that you have learned from reading this book. I hope that I have answered every question that you have on how to prevent and treat hair loss. I also hope that this has given you some knowledge on how to have a healthy hair and on how to maintain it.

I know that you might be suffering from hair loss right now, but always remember that it is never too late. You can always turn things around. With discipline and patience, you can achieve what you want in the near future.

Always remember that change would only start if you start acting. This book would be futile if you would not apply everything that is written here. I hope that you use and share everything that you have learned from this book.

Well then, go on and prevent that hair loss from happening. I wish you nothing but the best.

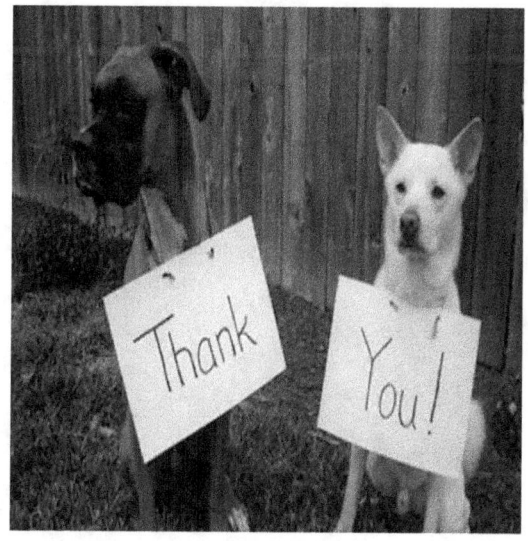

Finally, if you enjoyed this book, then I'd like to ask you for a favor, would you be kind enough to leave a review for this book on Amazon? It'd be greatly appreciated!

Thank you and good luck!